FAR OUT

Coloring for Adults

SANDRA TORK

"Far Out" Coloring for Adults takes you back to the Groovy 60's! Have fun and reminisce with "Far Out"! Color memories and revisit a unique and carefree time in life!

Crafted and Designed by Sandra Tork

with Light/Tork Productions

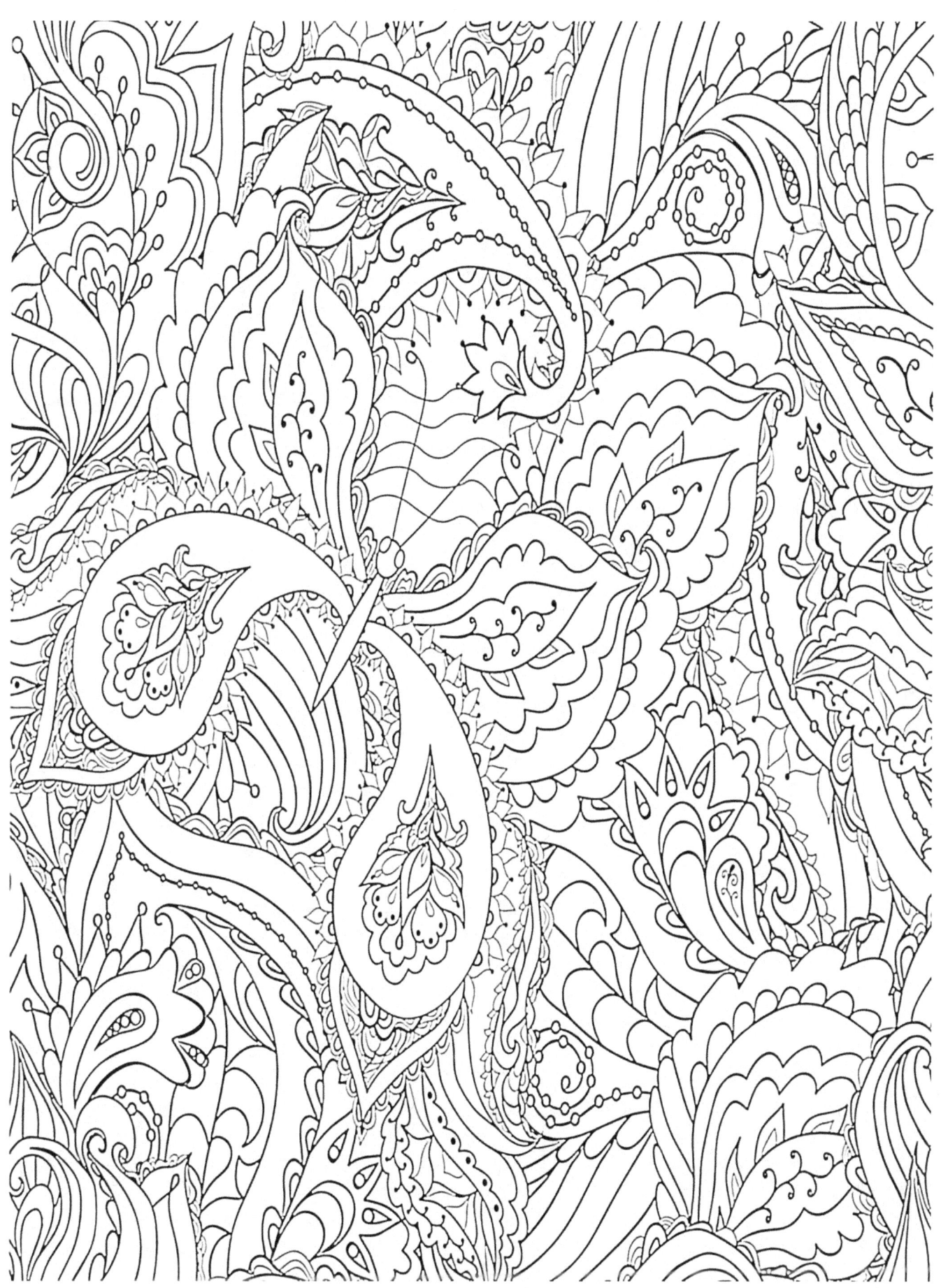

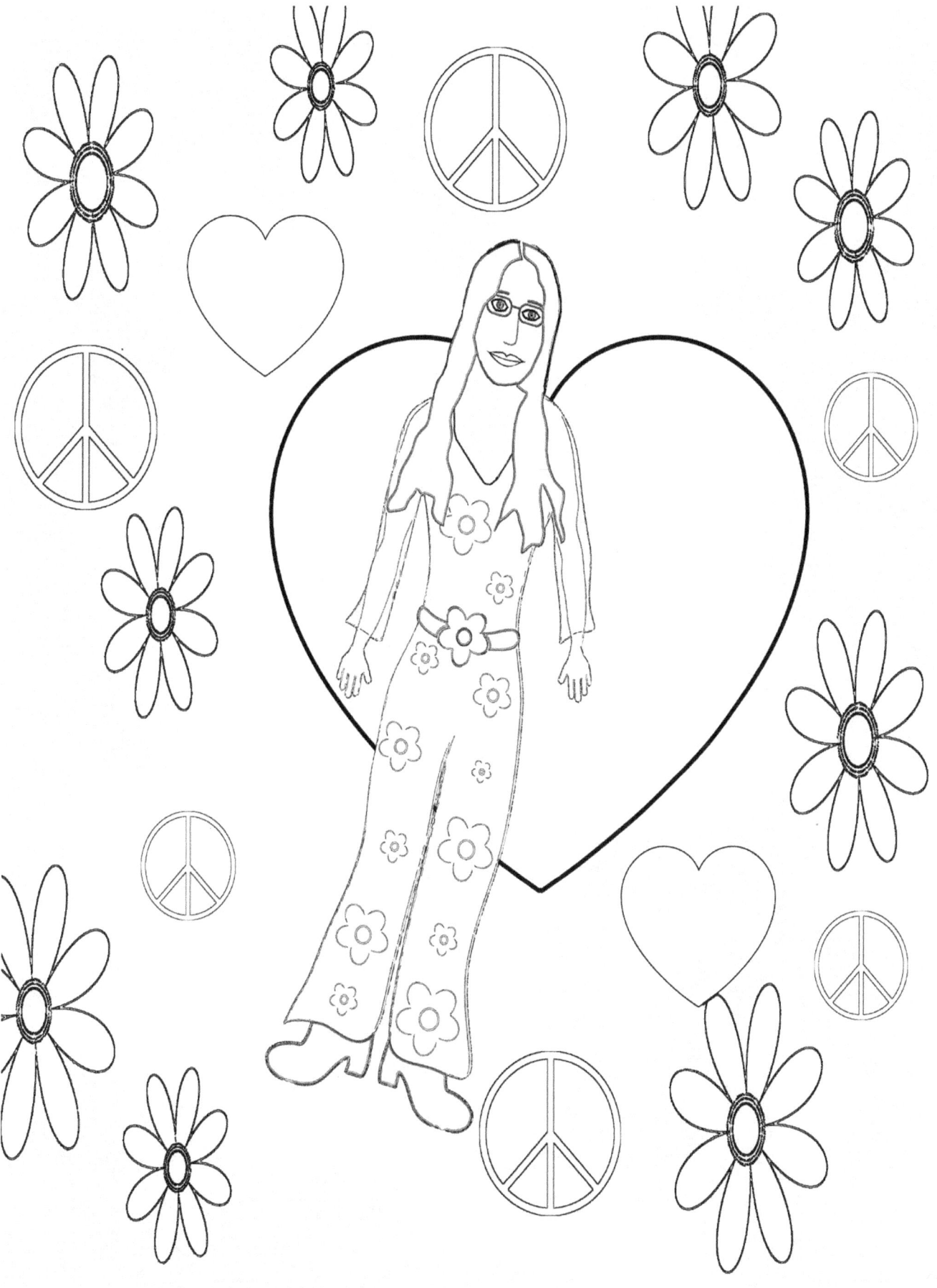

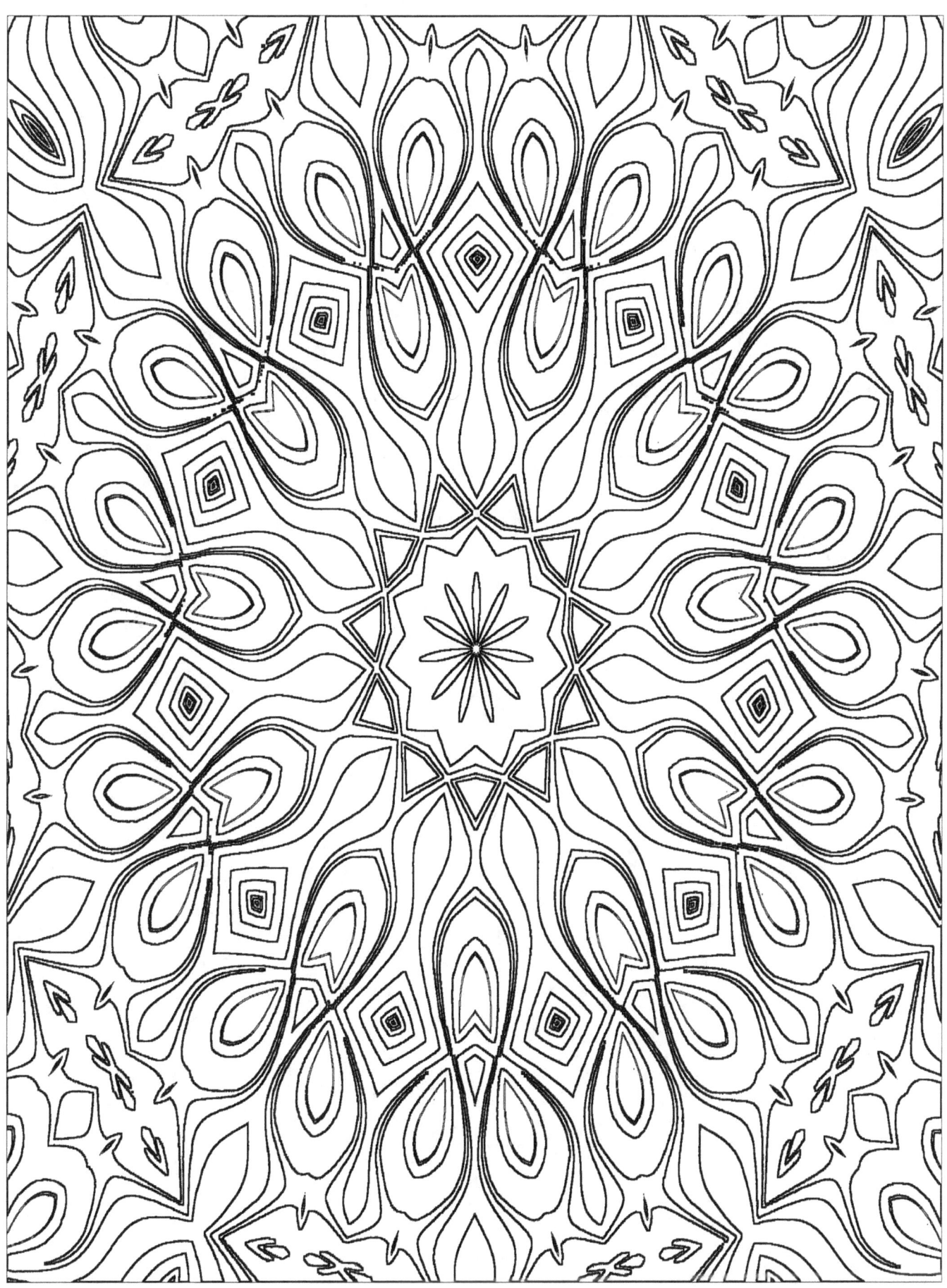

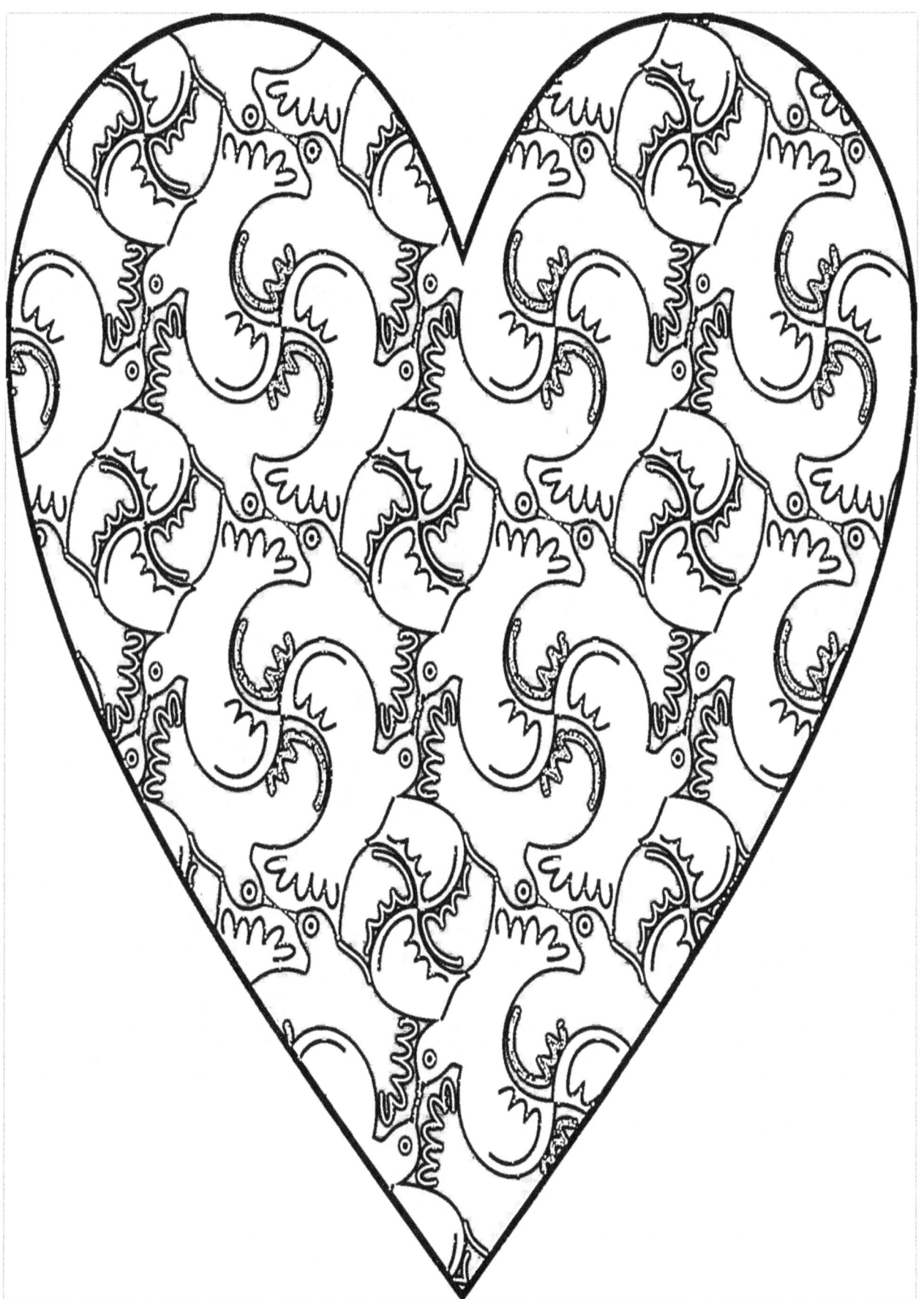

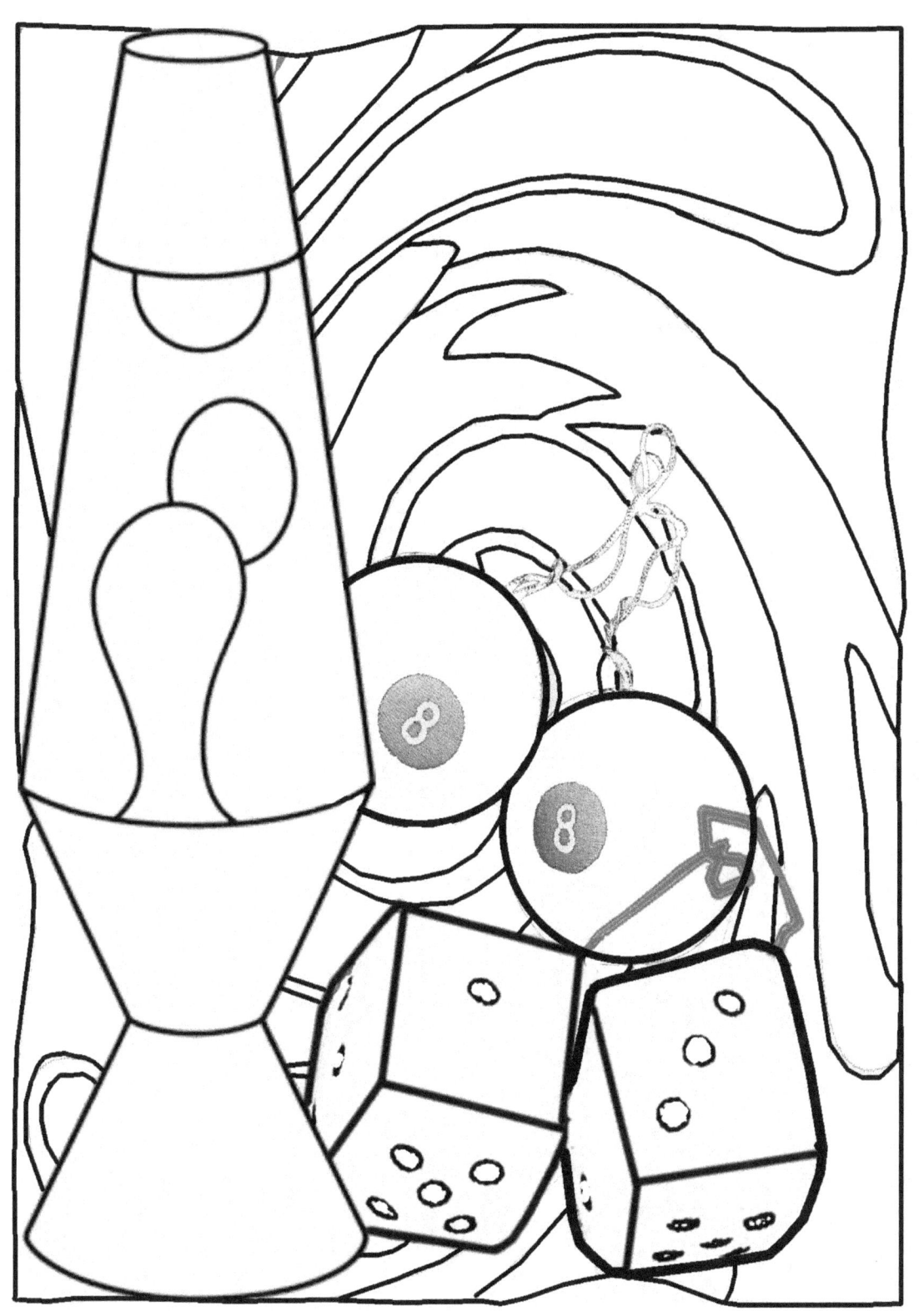

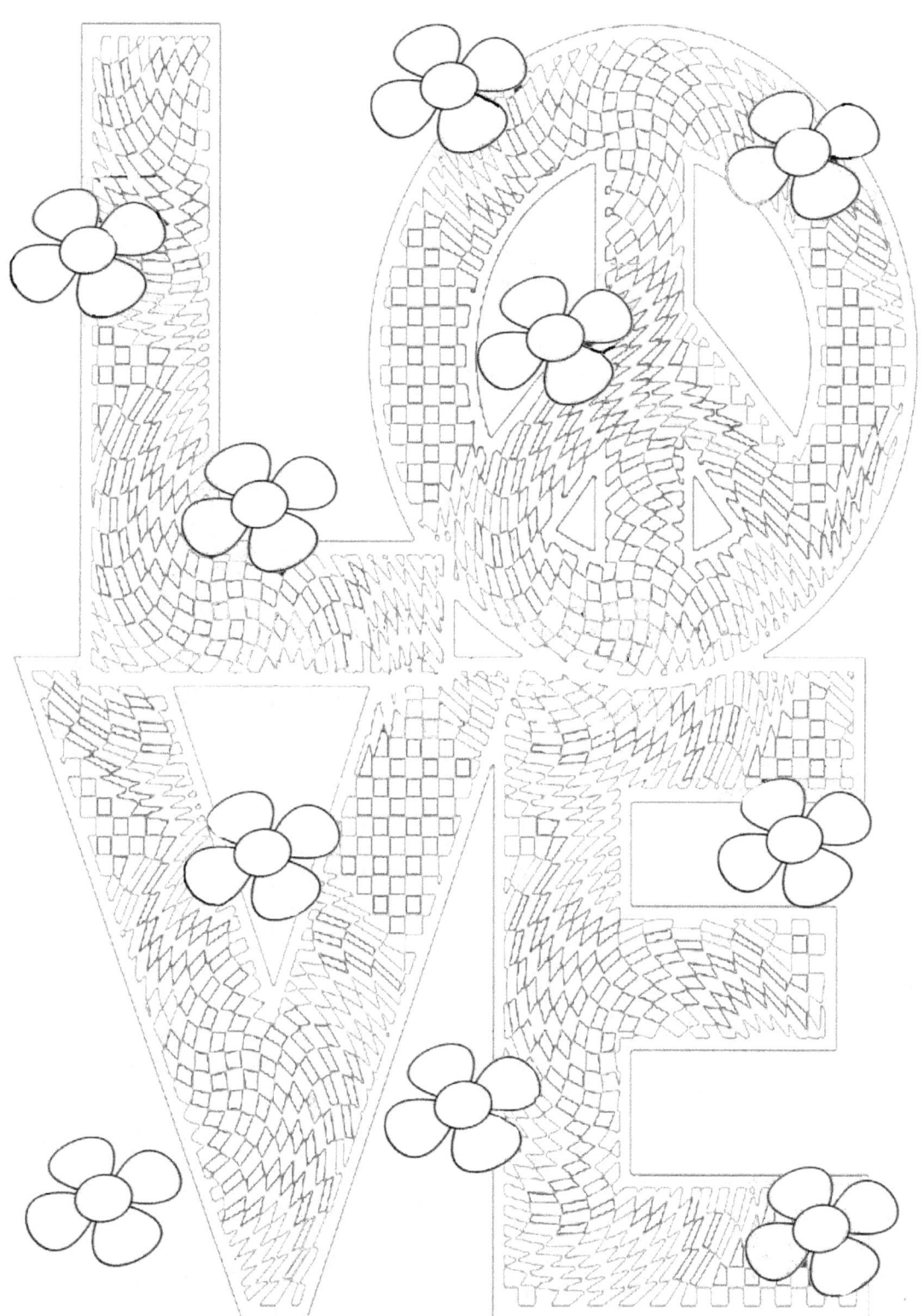

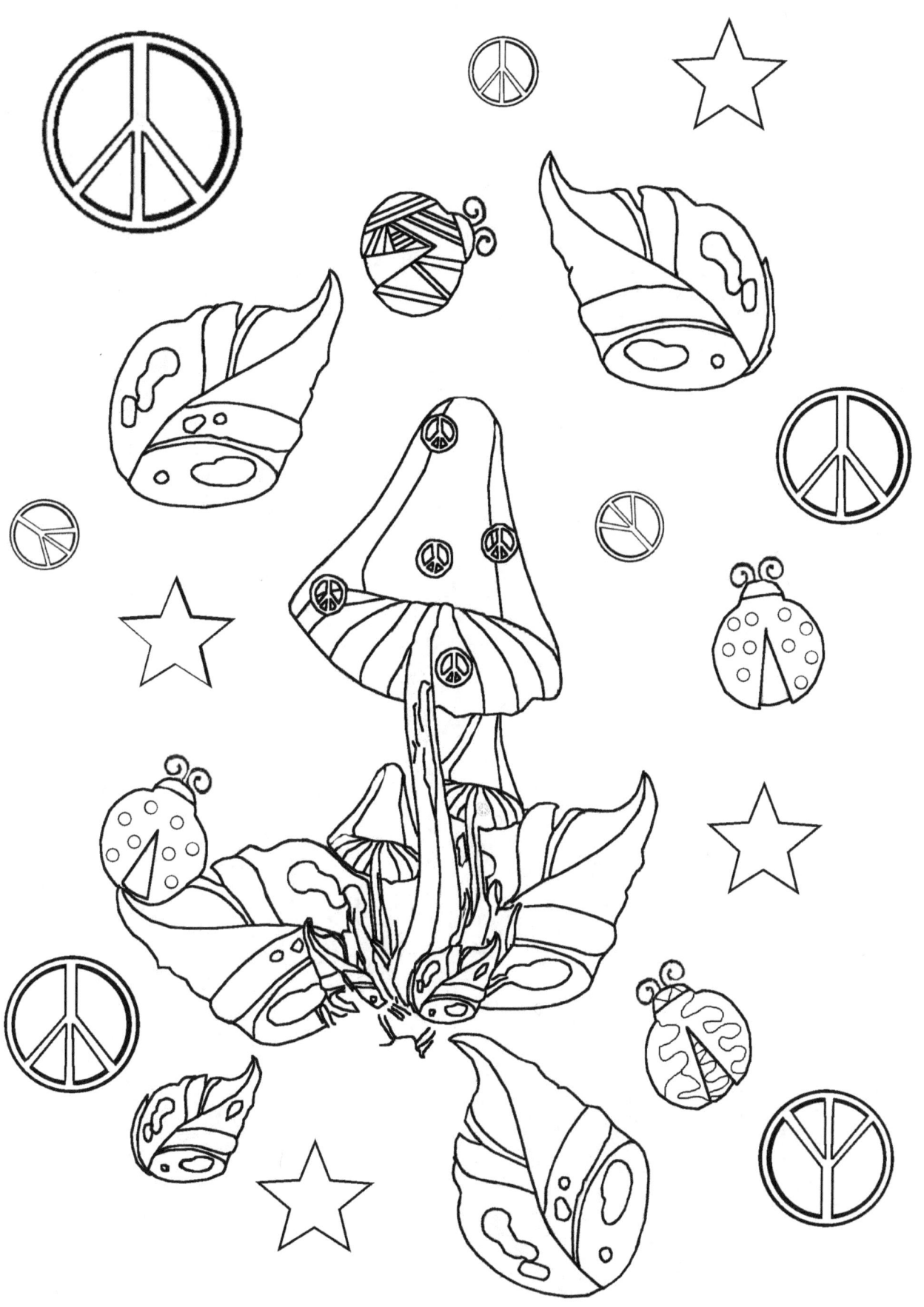

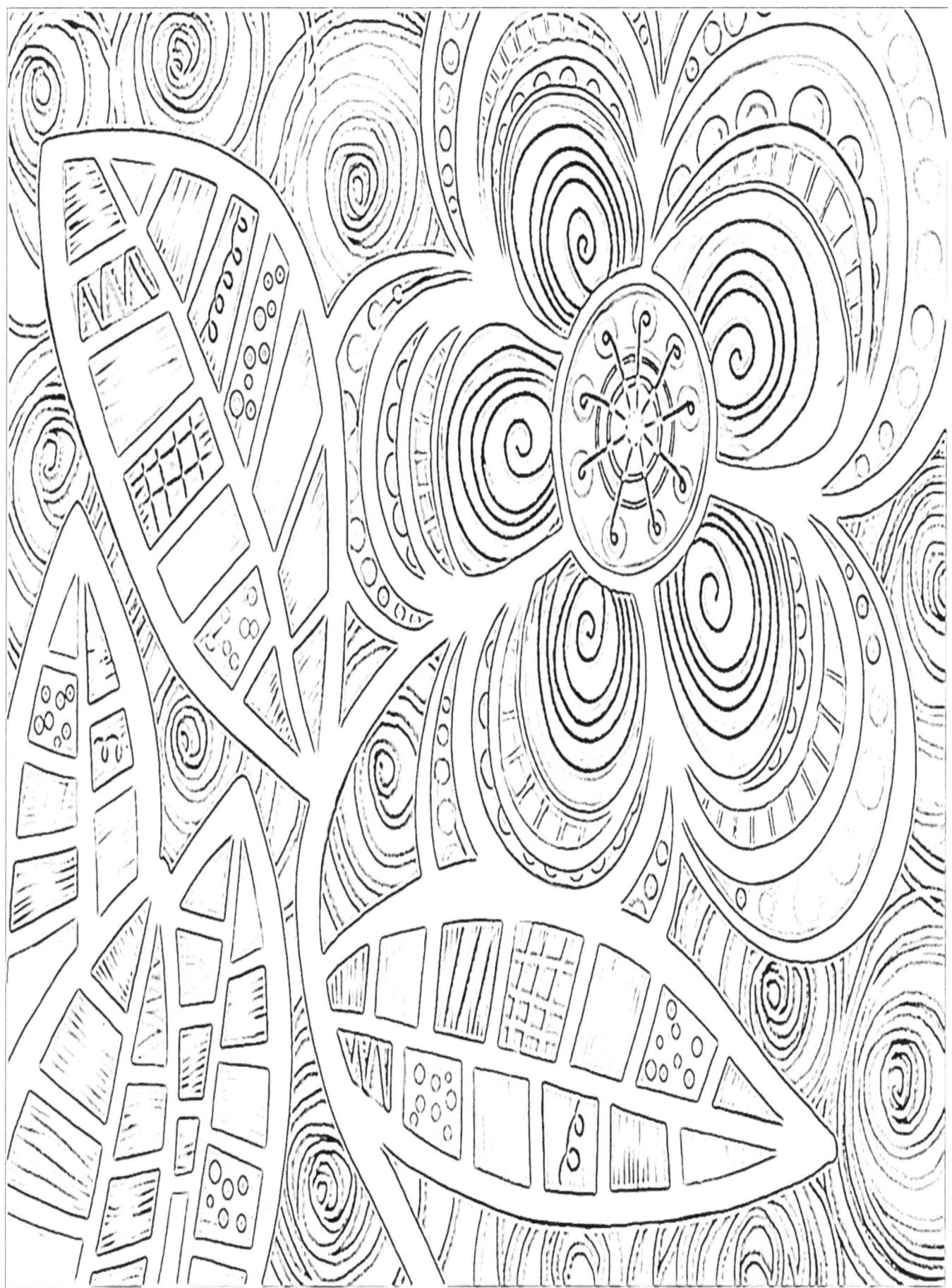

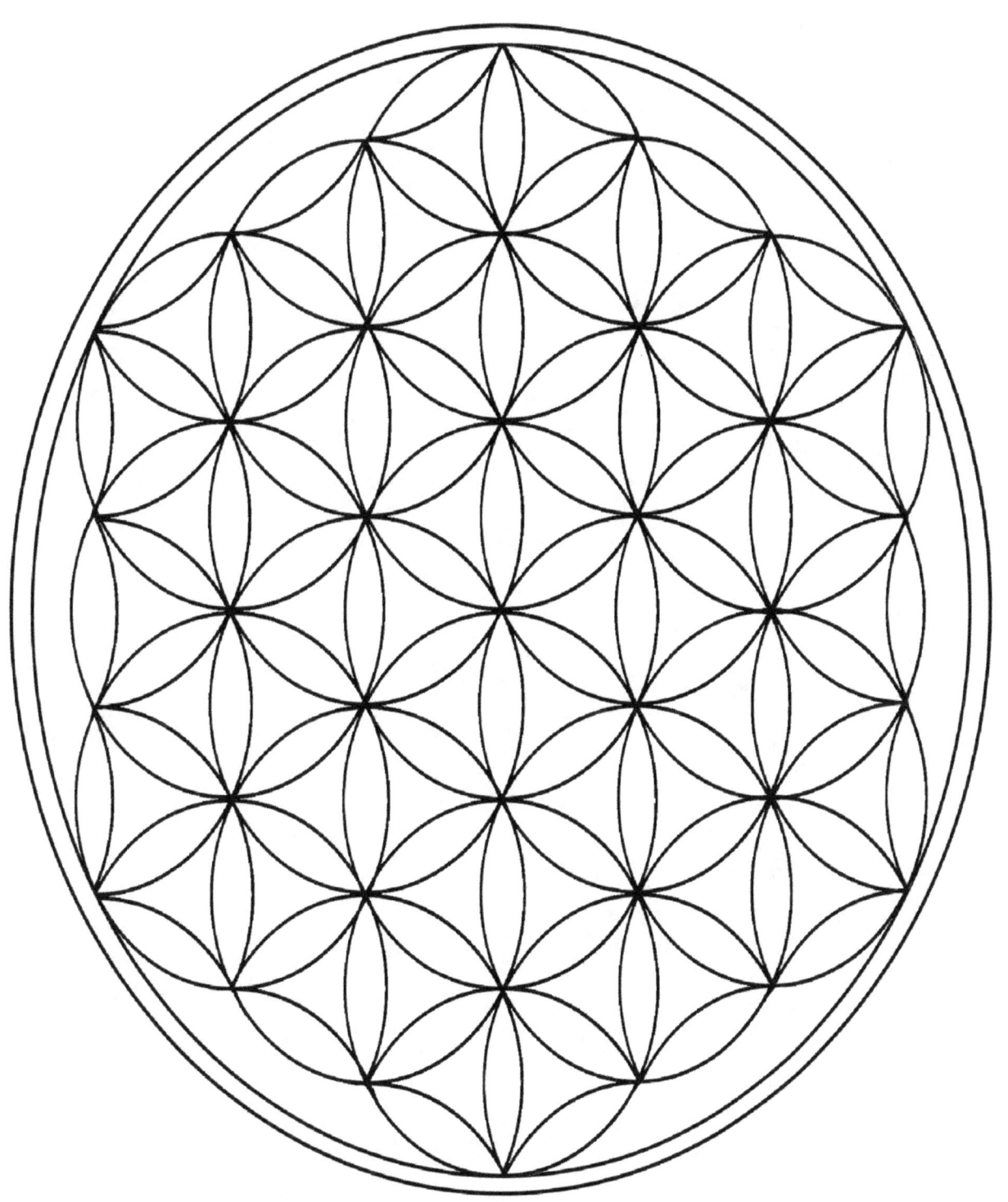

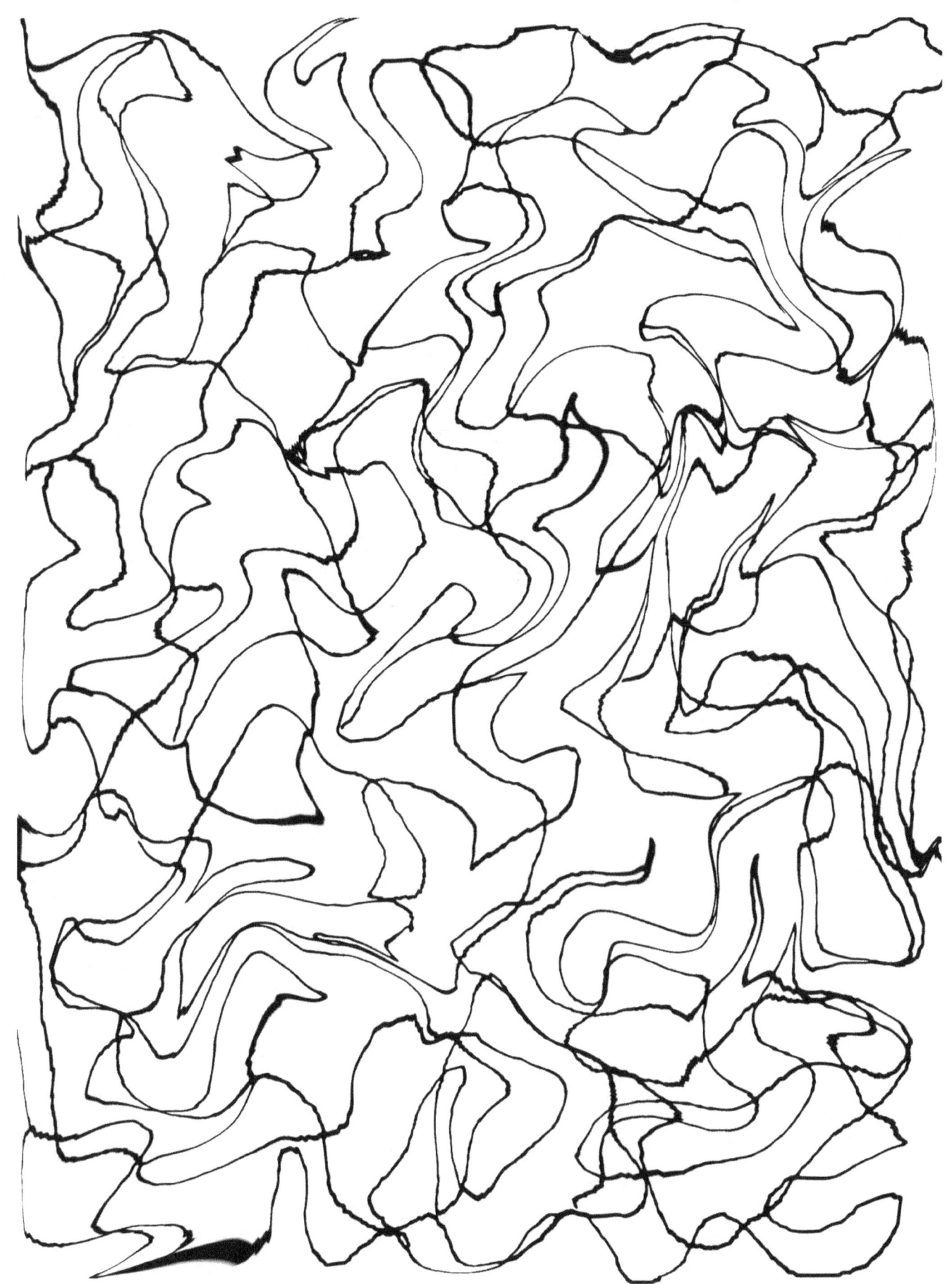

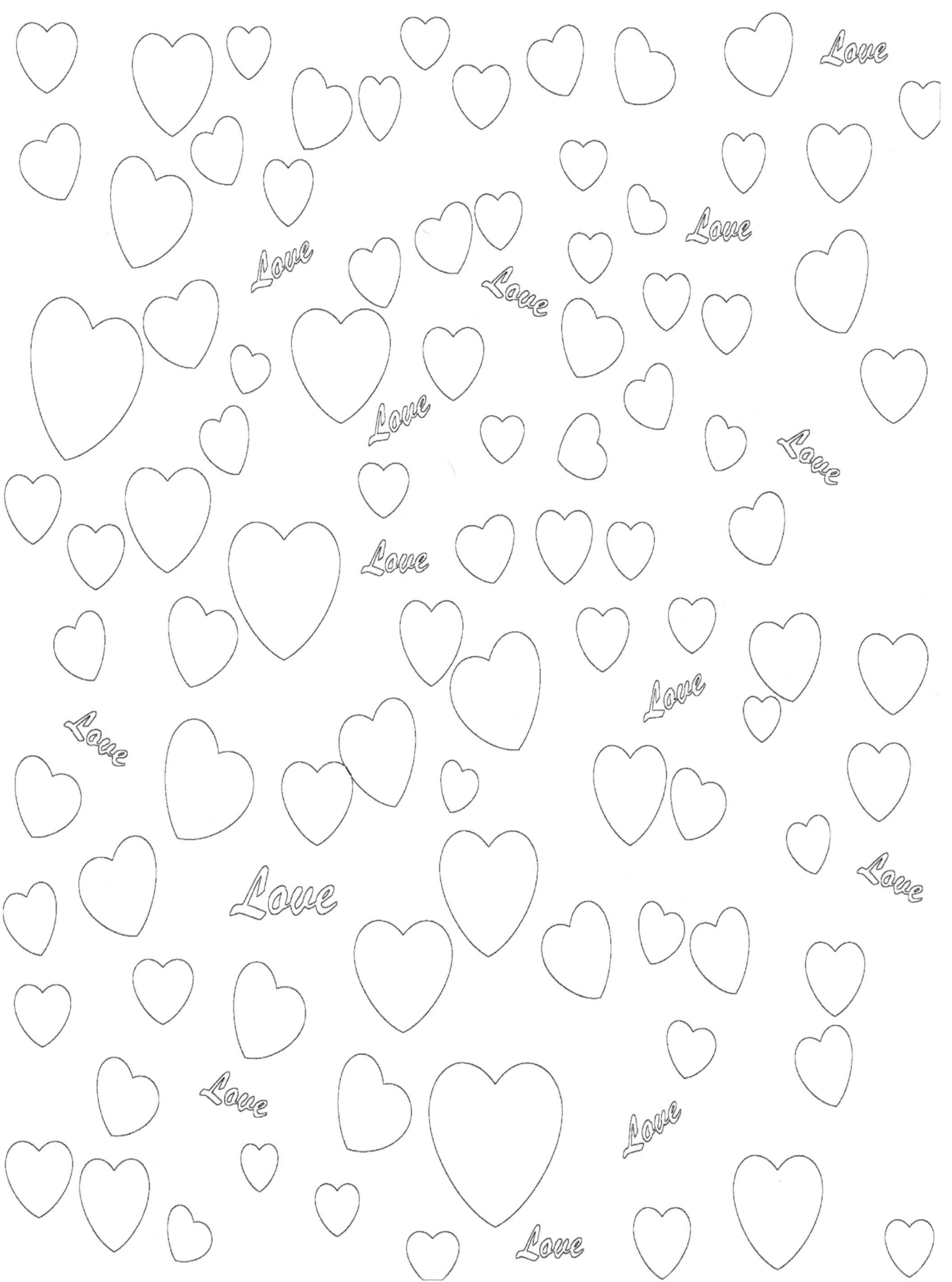

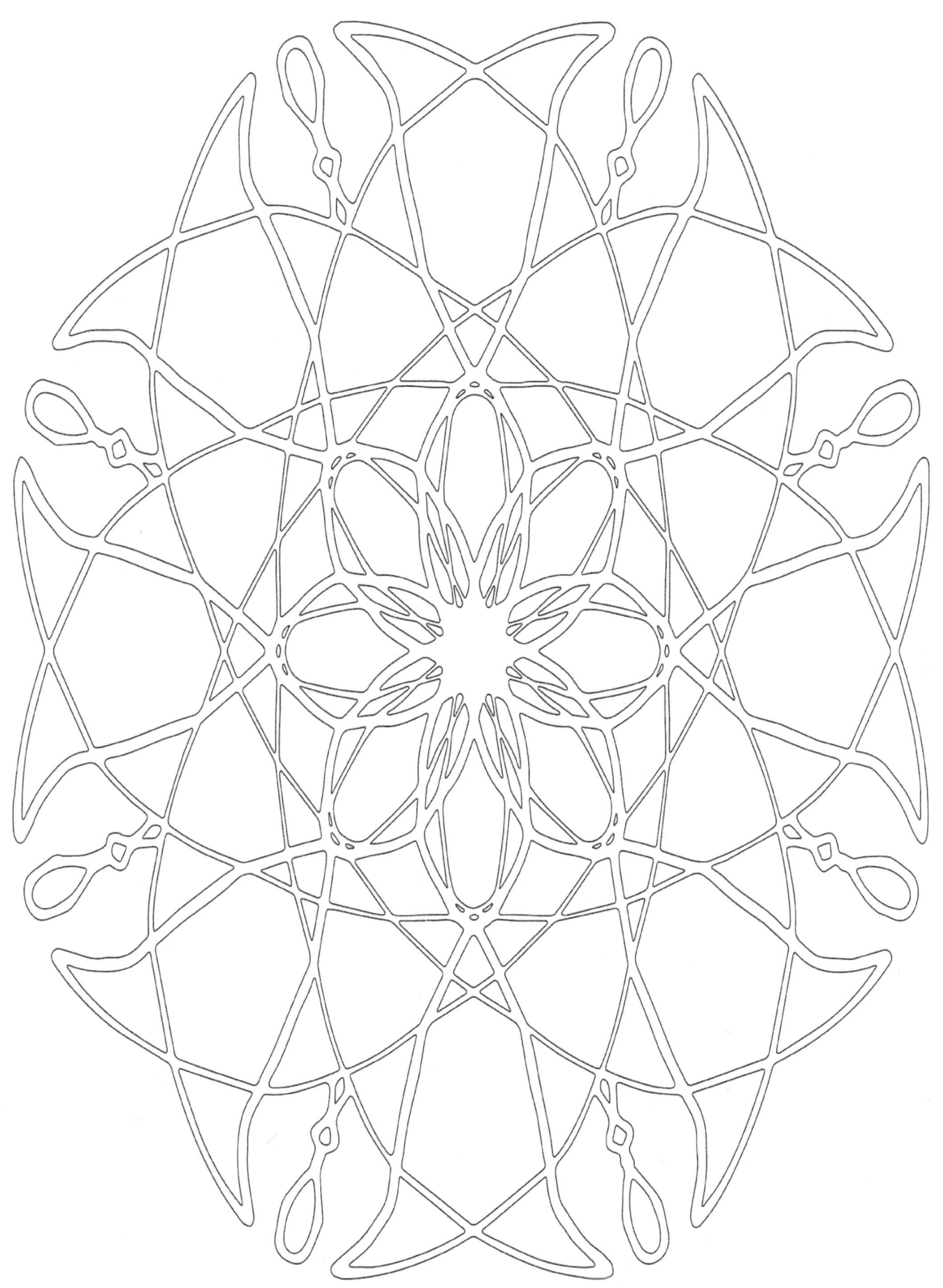

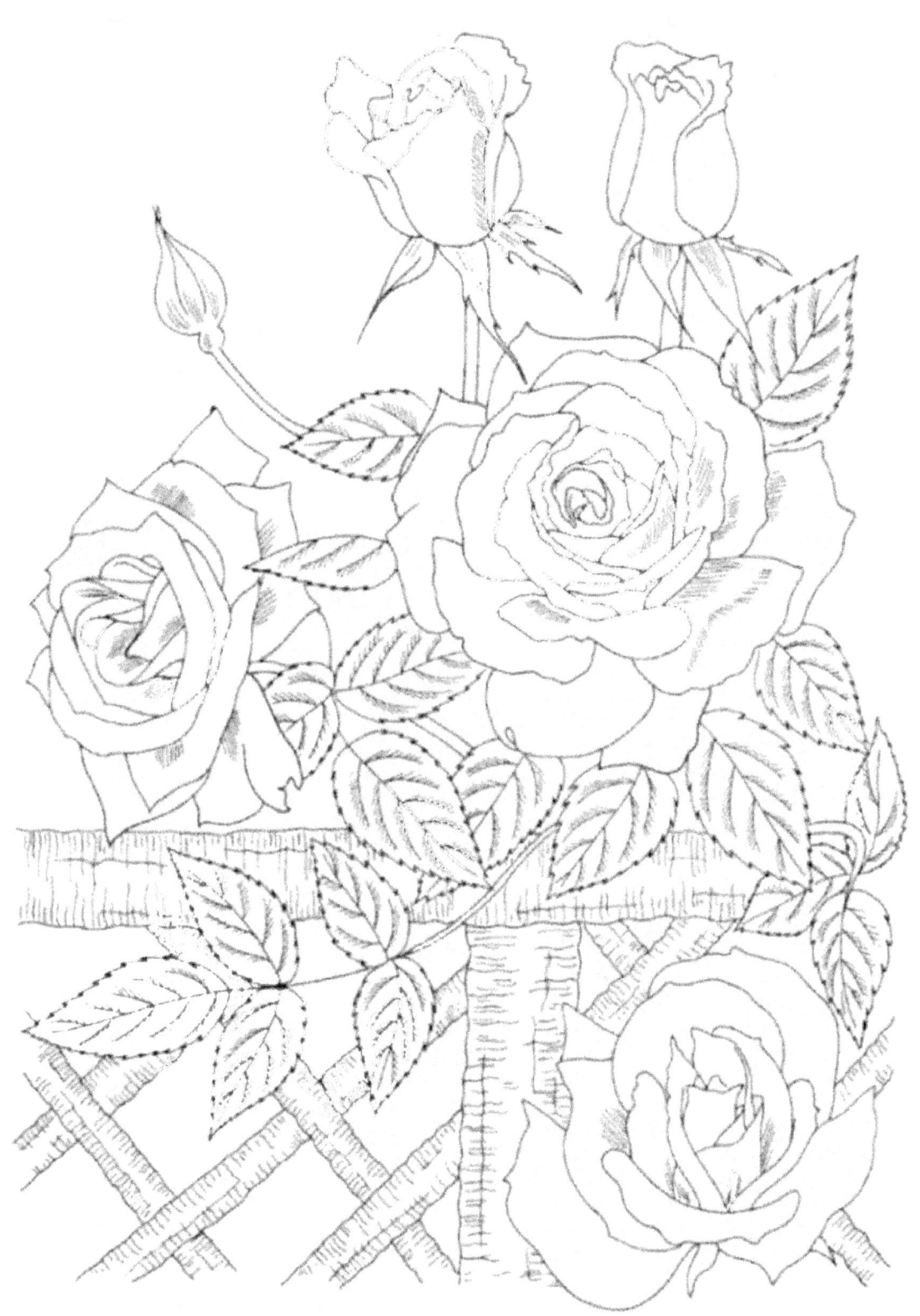

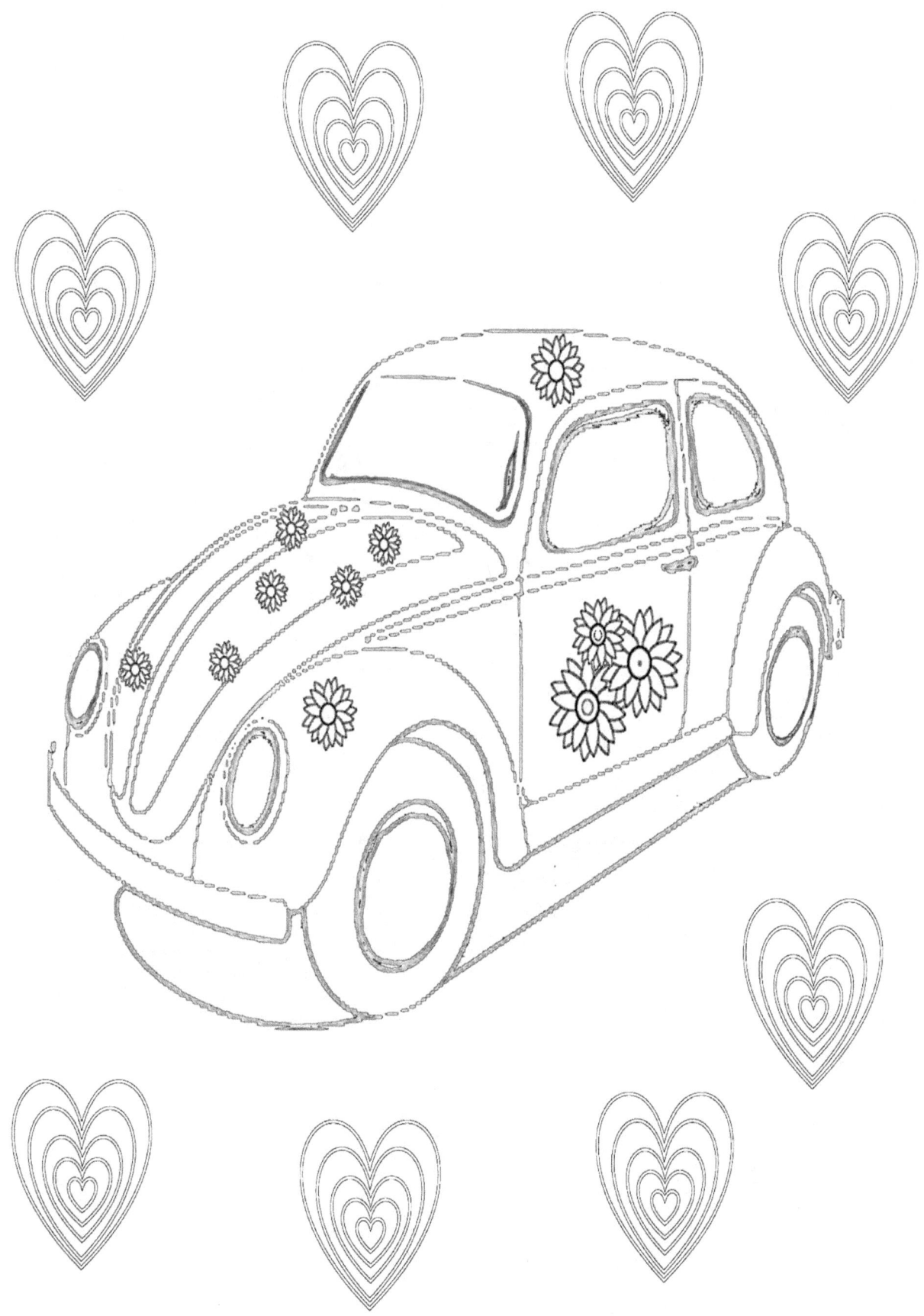

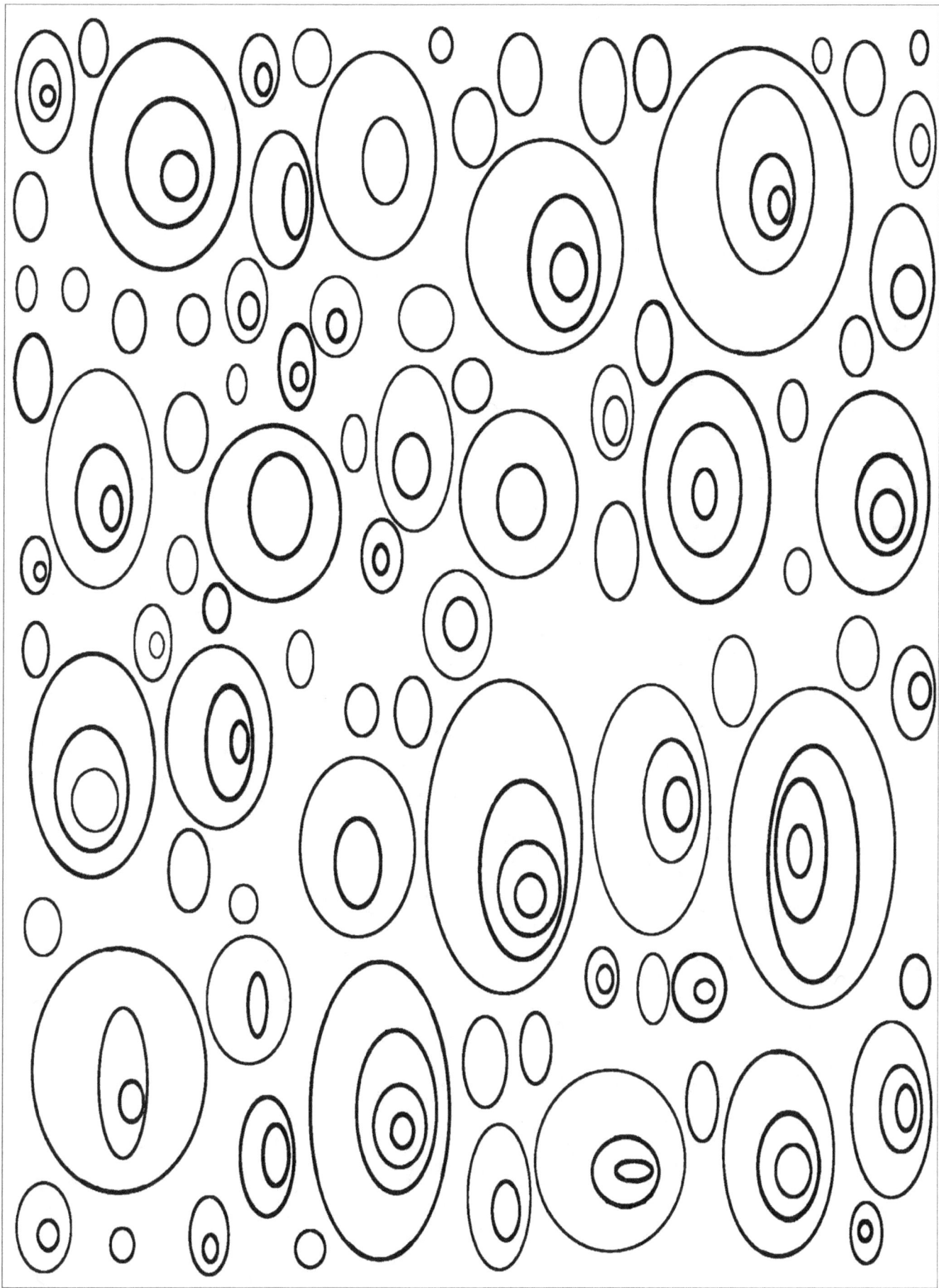

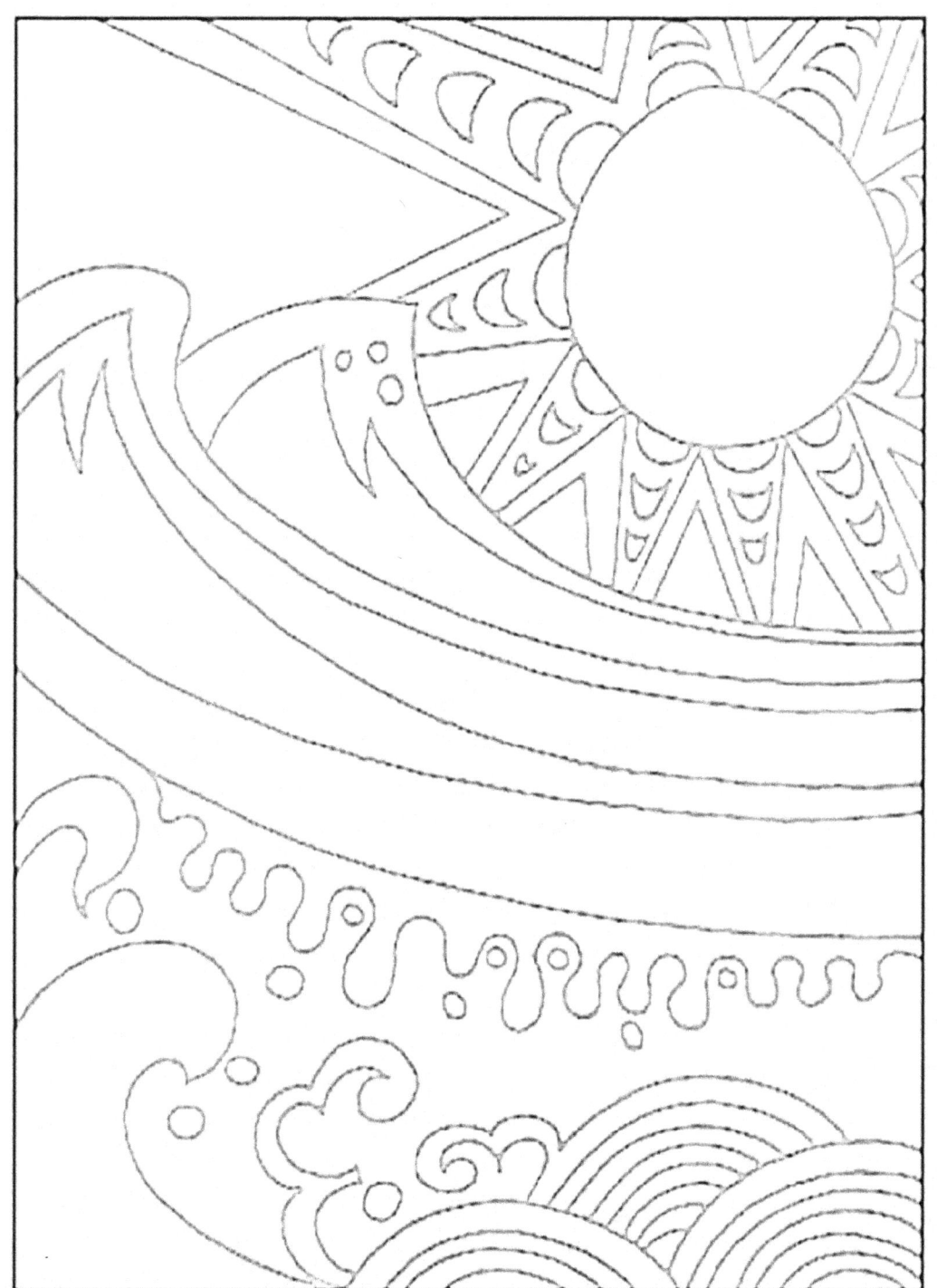

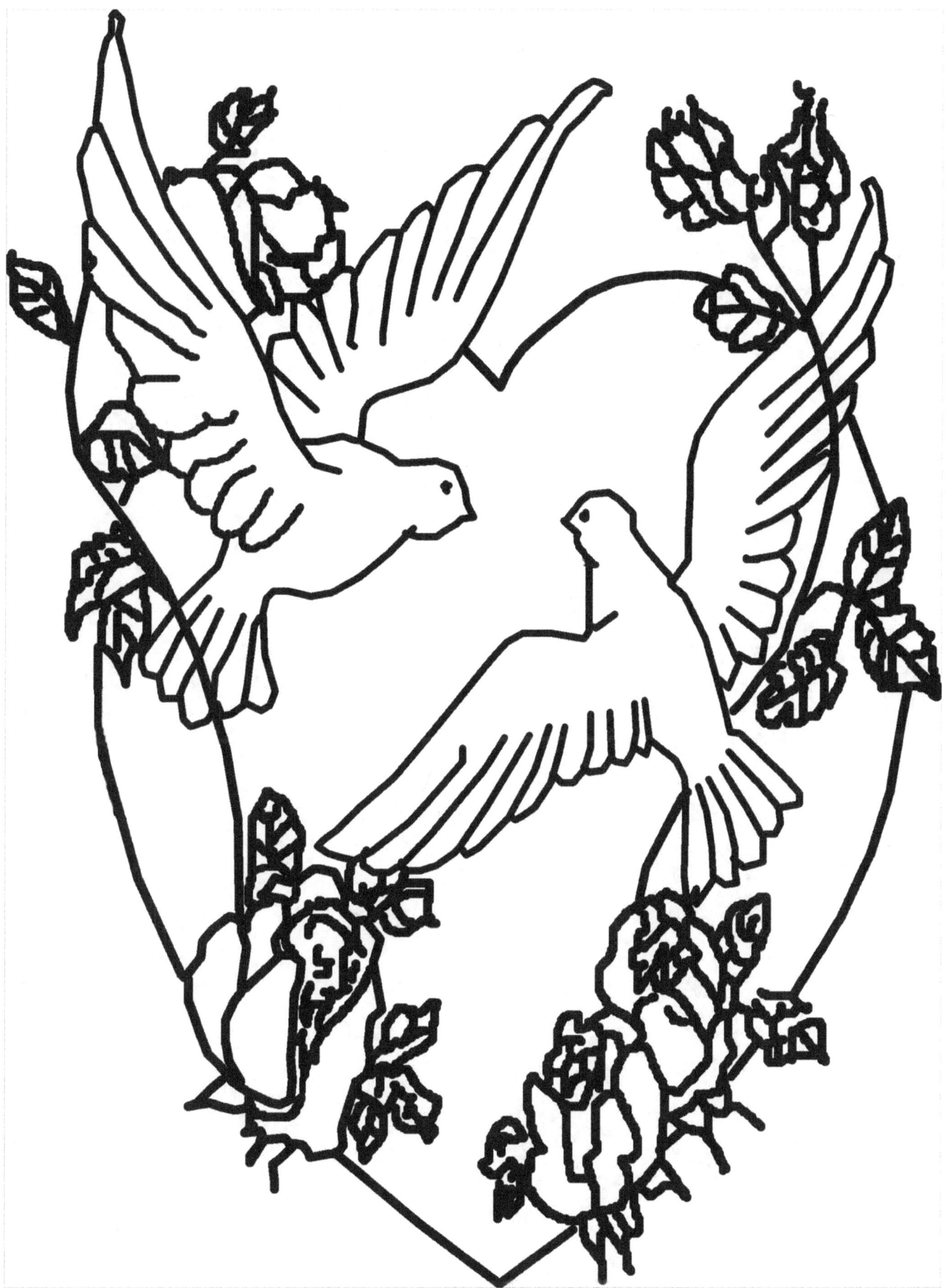

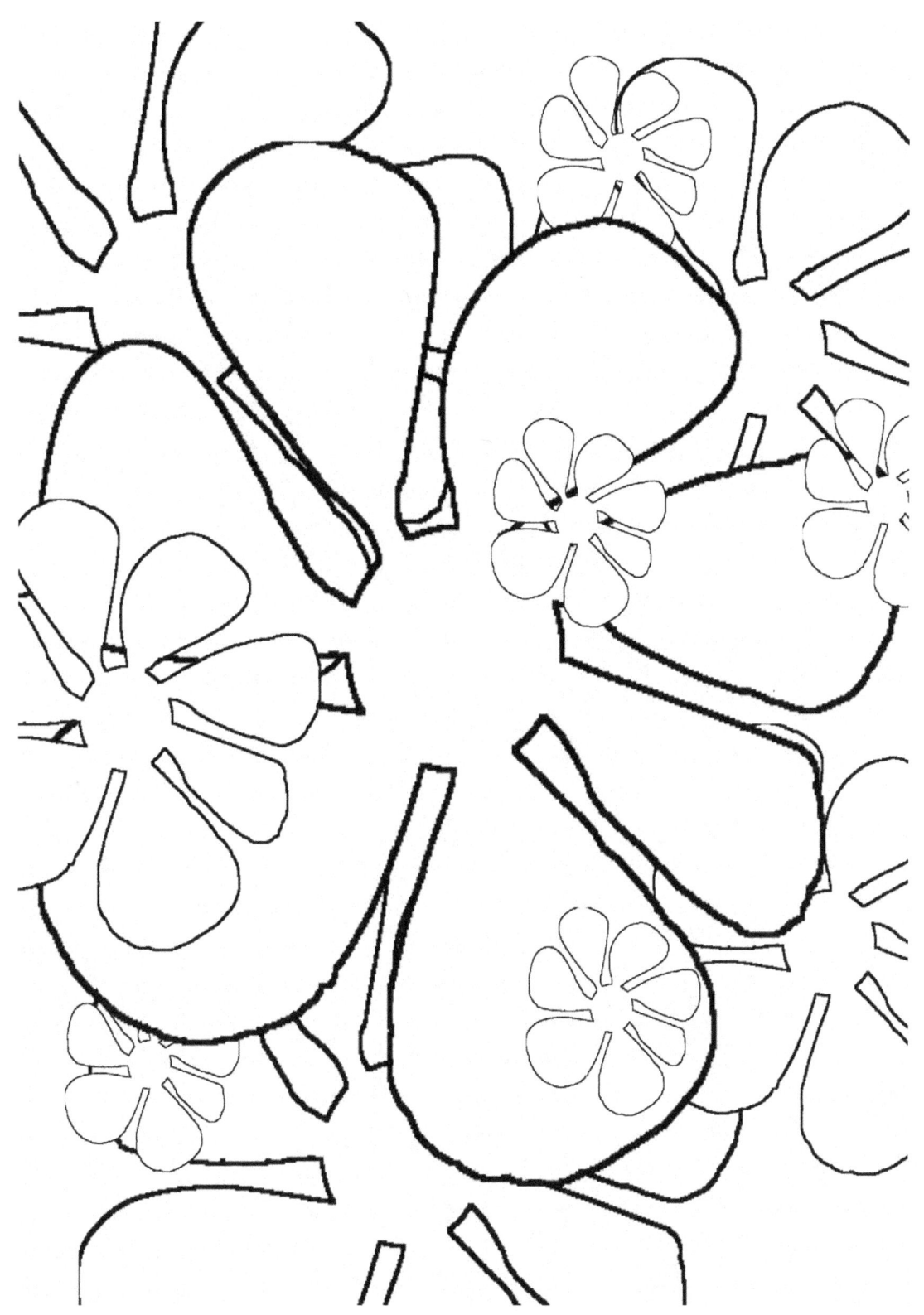

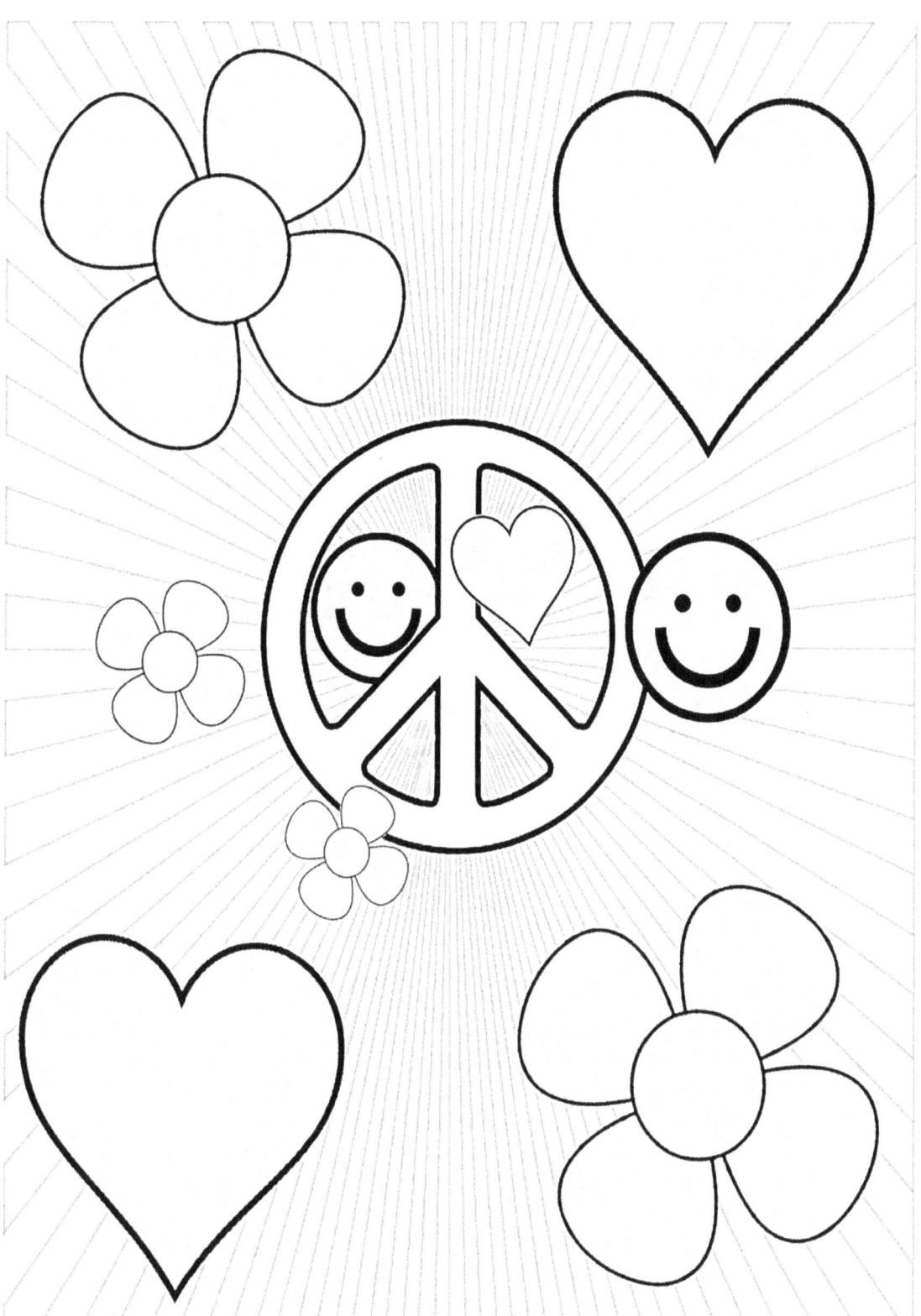

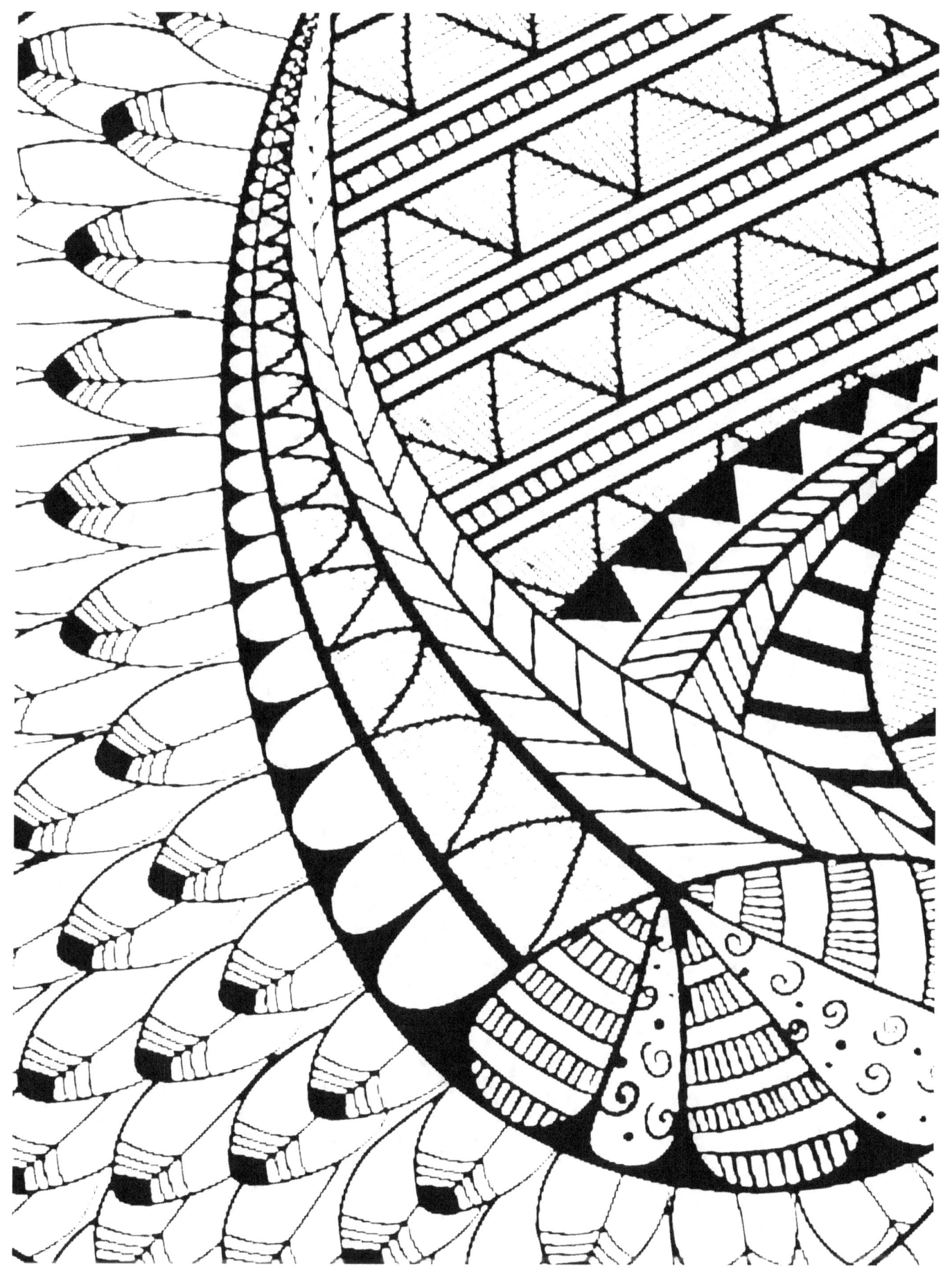

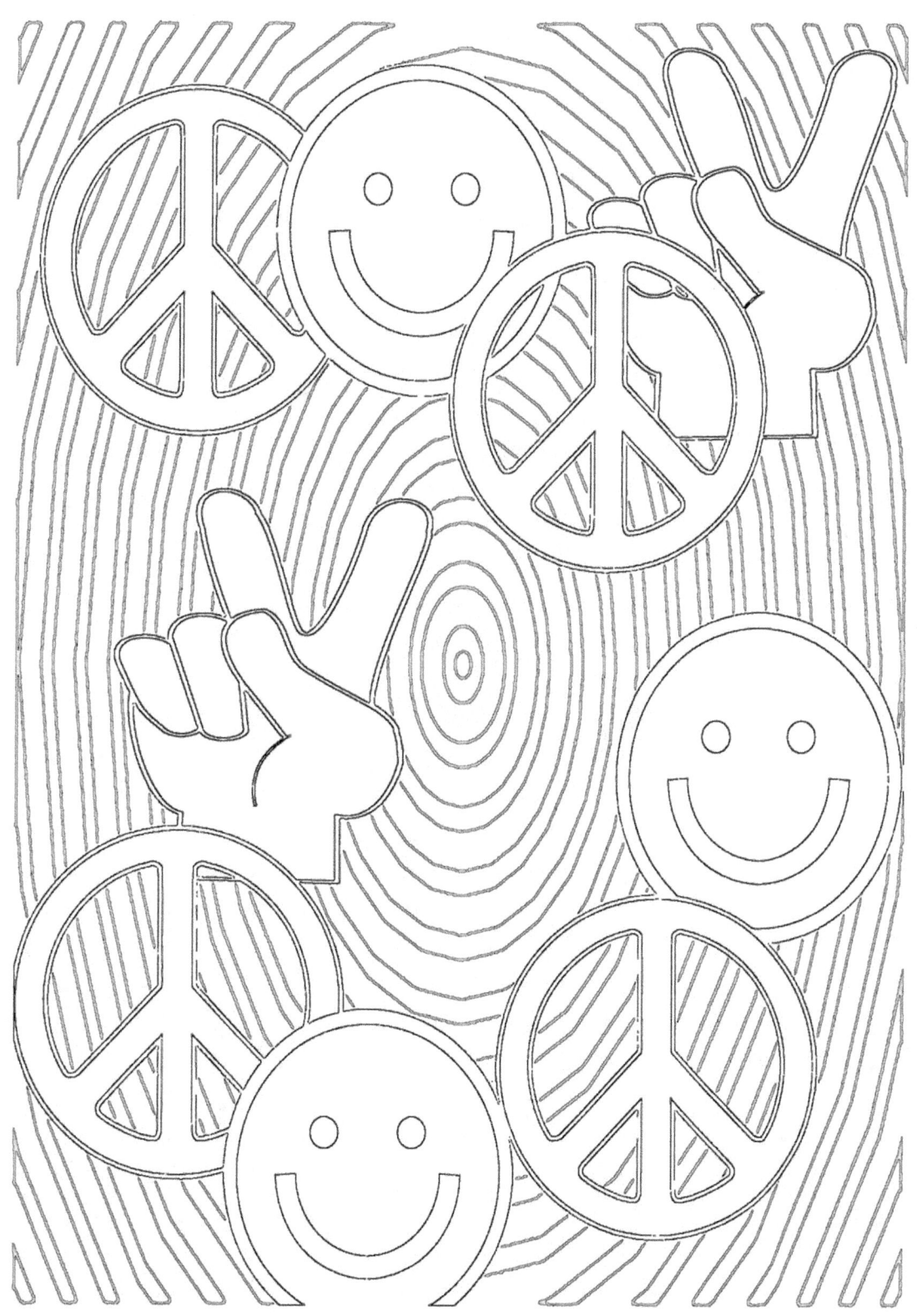

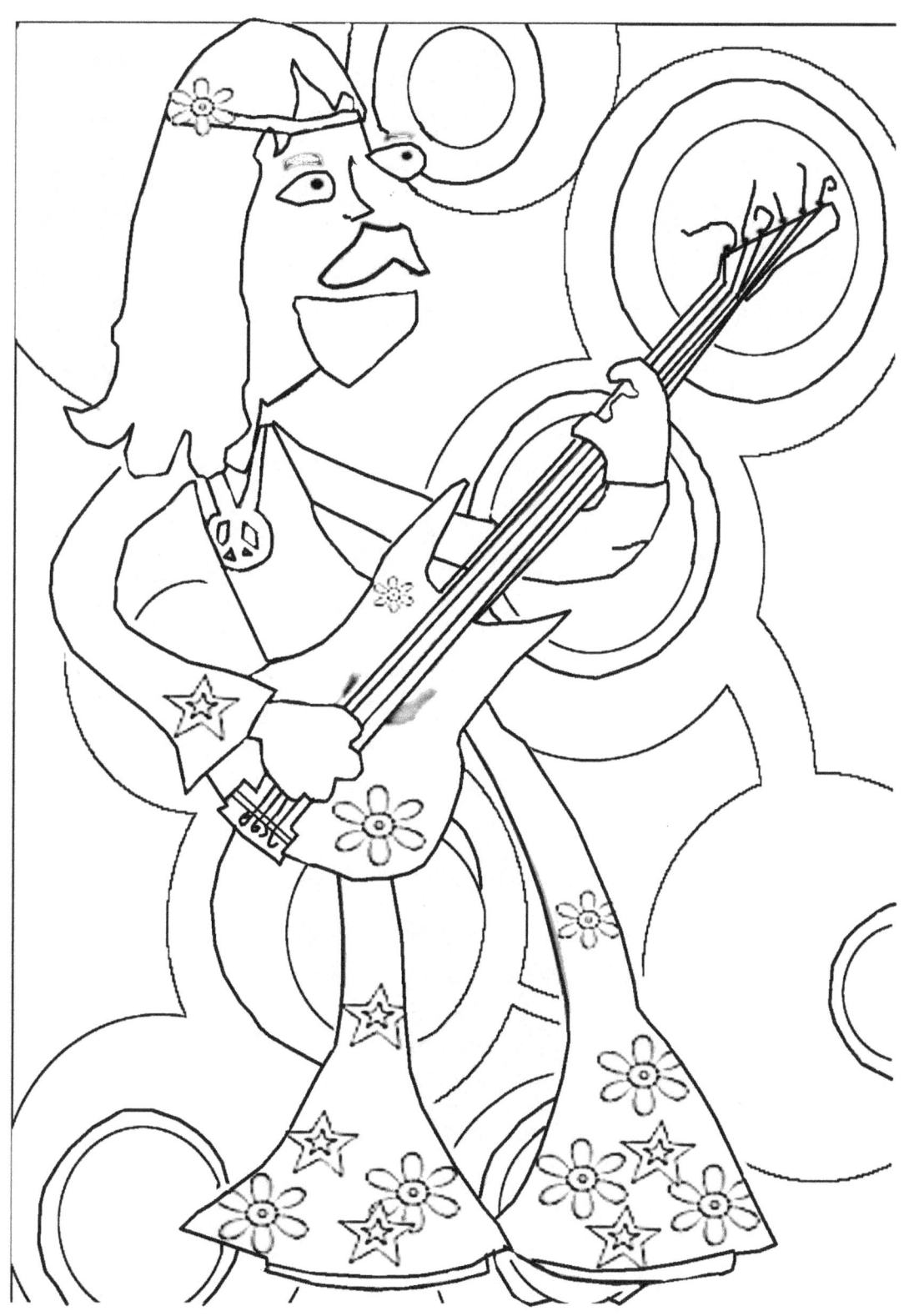

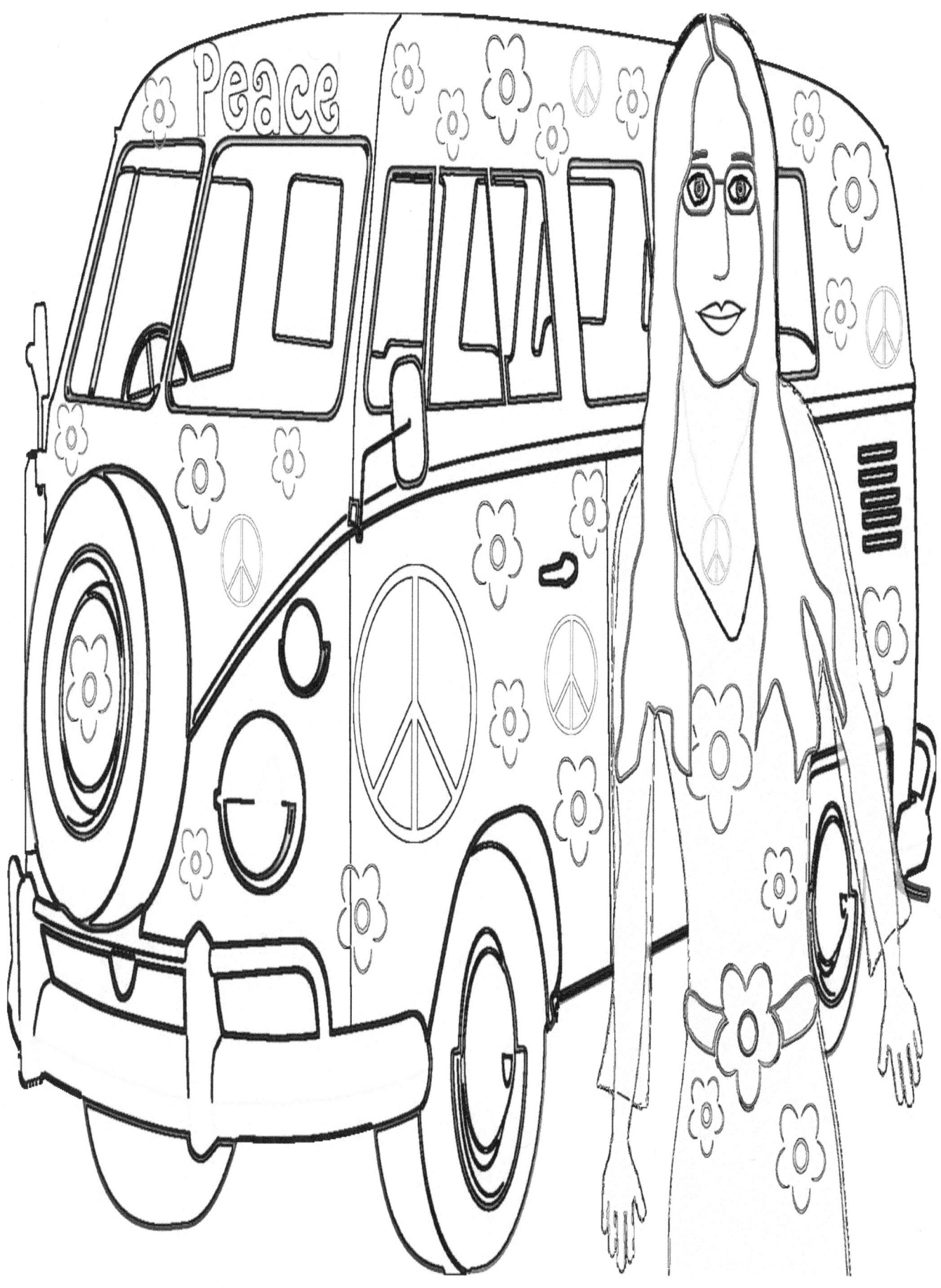

www.ingramcontent.com/pod-product-compliance
Lightning Source LLC
Chambersburg PA
CBHW081423280526
45788CB00009B/3206